Hypothyroid Diet Plan

A Beginner's Step-by-Step Guide to Reversing Fatigue, Unexplained Weight Gain, and Mind Fog: Includes Recipes and a 7-Day Meal Plan

mf

copyright © 2024 Brandon Gilta

All rights reserved No part of this book may be reproduced, or stored in a retrieval system, or transmitted in any form or by any means, electronic, mechanical, photocopying, recording, or otherwise, without express written permission of the publisher.

Disclaimer

By reading this disclaimer, you are accepting the terms of the disclaimer in full. If you disagree with this disclaimer, please do not read the guide.

All of the content within this guide is provided for informational and educational purposes only, and should not be accepted as independent medical or other professional advice. The author is not a doctor, physician, nurse, mental health provider, or registered nutritionist/dietician. Therefore, using and reading this guide does not establish any form of a physician-patient relationship.

Always consult with a physician or another qualified health provider with any issues or questions you might have regarding any sort of medical condition. Do not ever disregard any qualified professional medical advice or delay seeking that advice because of anything you have read in this guide. The information in this guide is not intended to be any sort of medical advice and should not be used in lieu of any medical advice by a licensed and qualified medical professional.

The information in this guide has been compiled from a variety of known sources. However, the author cannot attest to or guarantee the accuracy of each source and thus should not be held liable for any errors or omissions.

You acknowledge that the publisher of this guide will not be held liable for any loss or damage of any kind incurred as a result of this guide or the reliance on any information provided within this guide. You acknowledge and agree that you assume all risk and responsibility for any action you undertake in response to the information in this guide.

Using this guide does not guarantee any particular result (e.g., weight loss or a cure). By reading this guide, you acknowledge that there are no guarantees to any specific outcome or results you can expect.

All product names, diet plans, or names used in this guide are for identification purposes only and are the property of their respective owners. The use of these names does not imply endorsement. All other trademarks cited herein are the property of their respective owners.

Where applicable, this guide is not intended to be a substitute for the original work of this diet plan and is, at most, a supplement to the original work for this diet plan and never a direct substitute. This guide is a personal expression of the facts of that diet plan.

Where applicable, persons shown in the cover images are stock photography models and the publisher has obtained the rights to use the images through license agreements with third-party stock image companies.

Table of Contents

Introduction	**8**
What Is Hypothyroidism?	**10**
Causes of Hypothyroidism	11
Symptoms of Hypothyroidism	13
Medical Treatments for Hypothyroidism	14
Lifestyle Changes to Manage Hypothyroidism	16
What Is Hypothyroidism Diet?	**18**
Principles of Hypothyroidism Diet	18
Benefits of Hypothyroidism Diet	20
Disadvantages of Hypothyroidism Diet	21
5-Step Guide on How to Get Started with The Hypothyroidism Diet	**22**
Step 1: Engage Your Healthcare Provider	22
Step 2: Adopt a Balanced Diet	23
Step 3: Moderate Consumption of Foods that Can Disrupt Thyroid Function	25
Step 4: Prioritize Hydration and Regular Physical Activity	27
Step 5: Monitor Your Progress	28
Foods to Eat	30
Foods to Avoid	31
Sample Meal Plan	**34**
Day 1	34
Day 2	35
Day 3	36
Day 4	36
Day 5	37
Day 6	38
Day 7	39
Tips to Implement Your Meal Plan	40

Sample Recipes	**48**
Moroccan-Style Chicken	49
Green Monster Smoothie	51
Angel Hair Pasta	52
Greek-style hash with California Sweet Potatoes	53
Pistachio Salmon	55
Ginger-Chicken Noodle Soup	56
Smoky Stuffed Peppers	58
Kale Salad	61
Polish-Style Beet Soup	62
Brown Rice with Tomato and Avocado	64
Liver Detox Shake	65
Cheese Blintzes with Blackberries	66
English Tea	68
Roasted Chicken Breast	70
Butternut Squash with Cinnamon	72
Hearty Bean Soup	74
Conclusion	**76**
FAQ	**79**
References and Helpful Links	**81**

Introduction

If you're frequently fatigued, gaining weight inexplicably, or grappling with mood swings, hypothyroidism could be the cause. This condition, characterized by insufficient hormone production by the thyroid gland, affects millions globally and can significantly disrupt your life.

Managing hypothyroidism is possible, and it often begins with understanding the crucial role diet plays. Adjustments to your nutrition can help you regain energy, manage weight, and restore balance in your life.

Welcome to this comprehensive guide on diet for hypothyroidism. This comprehensive resource dives into nutrition's impact on thyroid health, highlighting foods that can stimulate thyroid function and those potentially detrimental. The aim isn't to promote a restrictive diet but to help you build a balanced, nutrient-rich eating plan that meets your specific needs.

To help you achieve this, this guide will help you:

- Realize the full extent of the impacts of hypothyroidism on your health and lifestyle;
- Understand the relationship between hypothyroidism and nutrition;
- Learn how to remove harmful elements from your body in preparation for the hypothyroidism diet;
- Refine your shopping list by listing down the important food items to eat, and the types of food to avoid;
- Create your own hypothyroidism meal plan;
- Lessen the effects of hypothyroidism on your health, and;
- Prepare and cook dishes that can boost the production of thyroid hormones.

This guide to nutrition for hypothyroidism is a resource for those seeking to take charge of their health. It provides insights into how diet can support thyroid function, nourish the body, and enhance overall vitality. By embracing a diet tailored to your needs, you're taking a significant step towards improved thyroid health and a symptom-free life. This journey towards understanding and managing hypothyroidism is your path toward optimal health.

What Is Hypothyroidism?

Hypothyroidism, or myxedema, is a lot more prevalent than you might assume. According to a recent study, about half of those suffering from this thyroid condition fail to recognize its signs and symptoms. They usually take note of it when they are already experiencing fatigue, rapid but unexplainable weight gain, and increased sensitivity to cold.

However, the impacts of hypothyroidism go deeper than these noticeable effects. Hormones produced by the thyroid gland are essential in:

- Regulating Metabolism: Thyroid hormones play a critical role in determining how your body uses energy, affecting almost every organ in your body.
- Heart Function: These hormones help control heart rate and blood pressure, impacting overall cardiovascular health.
- Digestion: Thyroid hormones can influence how your body processes food, potentially affecting digestion and nutrient absorption.

- Brain Development: Particularly important during infancy and childhood, thyroid hormones are crucial for normal brain and nervous system development.
- Bone Maintenance: They are involved in bone health, helping to regulate calcium levels in the body and maintain bone density.
- Body Temperature Regulation: Thyroid hormones help regulate body temperature, ensuring it stays at an optimal level for various bodily functions.

With such vital roles, it's no wonder that an underperforming thyroid can lead to a wide range of symptoms and health complications. That's why it's critical to understand the condition and how you can manage it effectively through your diet.

Causes of Hypothyroidism

If you've been diagnosed with hypothyroidism, you're not alone. This condition affects millions of people worldwide, and there are many possible causes. Some common causes include:

1. **Hashimoto's Thyroiditis:** This is an autoimmune disorder where the body's immune system mistakenly attacks the thyroid gland. The damage caused by this attack prevents the thyroid from producing enough hormones.

2. **Radiation Therapy:** Individuals who have undergone radiation therapy, especially for cancers of the neck and head, may experience hypothyroidism due to damage to the thyroid gland.
3. **Thyroid Surgery:** If part or all of the thyroid gland is removed during surgery, it can result in hypothyroidism. The remaining gland might not be able to produce enough thyroid hormone for the body's needs.
4. **Certain Medications:** Some medicines used for treating various conditions, including certain psychiatric, heart, and cancer medications, can sometimes affect the production of thyroid hormones.
5. **Iodine Deficiency:** Iodine is crucial for the production of thyroid hormones. A diet significantly low in iodine can cause hypothyroidism, particularly in regions where iodine levels in the soil and food supply are low.

By understanding the potential causes of your hypothyroidism, you can take steps to manage and improve your condition through a targeted diet plan. In the next section, we will discuss the symptoms of hypothyroidism, so you can better identify if this condition might be affecting your health.

Symptoms of Hypothyroidism

It's essential to recognize the signs and symptoms of hypothyroidism as early as possible. While some are noticeable, others can be more subtle but equally impactful on your overall health. Some common symptoms include:

1. **Fatigue**: Hypothyroidism can cause extreme tiredness, making it difficult to perform daily activities or stay alert.
2. **Sensitivity to Cold**: People with hypothyroidism often feel unusually cold due to slowed metabolism affecting body temperature regulation.
3. **Constipation**: Slowed digestive function can lead to constipation, a common symptom of hypothyroidism.
4. **Dry Skin**: Hypothyroidism can decrease sweating, leading to dry, flaky skin and sometimes an unusually pale appearance.
5. **Weight Gain**: Unexplained weight gain can occur as the slowed metabolism reduces the body's calorie-burning capability.
6. **Puffy Face**: Fluid retention, a potential effect of hypothyroidism, can lead to facial puffiness.
7. **Hoarseness**: Swelling in the thyroid can put pressure on the voice box, causing a hoarse or raspy voice.
8. **Elevated Blood Cholesterol Level**: Hypothyroidism can raise the level of low-density lipoprotein (LDL) cholesterol in the blood.

9. **Muscle Weakness and Aches**: Hypothyroidism can cause muscle weakness, tenderness, stiffness, and aching.
10. **Depression**: Due to the overall physical discomfort and fatigue, individuals with hypothyroidism may experience depression.
11. **Impaired Memory**: Some people might experience forgetfulness or difficulty concentrating, often referred to as "brain fog."
12. **Slowed Heart Rate**: The lack of thyroid hormone can slow the heart rate, making it harder for the heart to pump blood.
13. **Hair Loss**: Hair can become brittle and fall out because of the changes in metabolism and nutrient absorption.
14. **Menstrual Changes**: Women may experience heavier, longer periods or increased frequency of menstruation.

If you are experiencing any of these symptoms, it's essential to consult with your healthcare provider for proper diagnosis and treatment.

Medical Treatments for Hypothyroidism

Hypothyroidism is a manageable condition with several treatment options available. The approach to treatment is often tailored to the individual's needs, but commonly includes:

1. **Hormone Replacement Therapy**: This is the most common treatment for hypothyroidism. It involves daily use of the synthetic thyroid hormone levothyroxine. This oral medication restores adequate hormone levels, reversing the signs and symptoms of hypothyroidism.
2. **Regular Monitoring**: After starting hormone replacement therapy, doctors will require regular blood tests to monitor thyroid function. Based on these results, they may adjust the dosage of medication to ensure optimal treatment.
3. **Dietary Modifications**: While not a standalone treatment, dietary changes can support thyroid health. Consuming a balanced diet rich in iodine and selenium can aid in hormone production.
4. **Treatment of Underlying Conditions**: If hypothyroidism is caused by an underlying condition, such as an autoimmune disease or certain types of medication, treating that condition can help manage hypothyroidism symptoms.
5. **Lifestyle Changes**: Regular exercise, sufficient sleep, and stress management techniques can help manage symptoms and improve overall well-being in individuals with hypothyroidism.

With proper treatment and management, individuals with hypothyroidism can lead healthy and fulfilling lives.

Lifestyle Changes to Manage Hypothyroidism

Managing hypothyroidism often involves making certain lifestyle changes to help control symptoms and improve overall health. These changes can complement medical treatments and include:

1. **Healthy Eating**: Consuming a balanced diet rich in fruits, vegetables, lean proteins, and whole grains can provide the nutrients necessary for thyroid health. Avoiding excess iodine and soy is often recommended.
2. **Regular Exercise**: Engaging in regular physical activity can boost energy levels, combat fatigue, and help maintain a healthy weight. It's important to choose an exercise regime that suits one's fitness level.
3. **Adequate Sleep**: Ensuring sufficient sleep can help manage fatigue, a common symptom of hypothyroidism. Establishing a regular sleep schedule can be beneficial.
4. **Stress Management**: Techniques such as yoga, meditation, and deep breathing exercises can help manage stress, which can exacerbate hypothyroid symptoms.
5. **Regular Check-ups**: Regular medical check-ups are essential to monitor thyroid hormone levels and adjust treatment as necessary.

6. **Avoid Certain Foods and Supplements**: Some foods and supplements might interfere with thyroid hormone absorption. These include high-fiber foods, iron, calcium, and certain antacids containing aluminum hydroxide.
7. **Limiting Intake of Goitrogens**: Goitrogens are substances that interfere with the way the body uses iodine. They are found in certain foods like broccoli, cabbage, and kale. Cooking these foods can inactivate the goitrogens.
8. **No Smoking**: Tobacco smoke has substances that affect the thyroid gland and may influence the severity of hypothyroidism symptoms.
9. **Moderate Alcohol Consumption**: High alcohol intake can have an adverse effect on thyroid function and can interfere with the effectiveness of medication.

By implementing these lifestyle changes, individuals with hypothyroidism can better manage their condition and improve their overall health.

What Is Hypothyroidism Diet?

A healthy diet is crucial for maintaining overall health and well-being, but it can be especially beneficial for individuals with hypothyroidism. A hypothyroidism diet focuses on consuming nutrient-dense foods that support thyroid function and minimize symptoms.

Principles of Hypothyroidism Diet

The principles of a Hypothyroidism Diet are based on consuming nutrient-dense foods that support thyroid function and overall health. These principles include:

1. **Eating Whole Foods**: A diet rich in whole foods such as fruits, vegetables, lean proteins, and healthy fats is beneficial for those with hypothyroidism.
2. **Including Thyroid-Supportive Nutrients**: Consuming foods high in zinc, selenium, omega-3s, and iodine can help improve thyroid function.
3. **Balanced Plate Concept**: This involves filling 50% of your plate with non-starchy vegetables, and 25% with lean protein.

4. **Limiting Foods That Interfere With Thyroid Function**: Certain foods may interfere with thyroid hormone absorption or production and should be limited.
5. **Consuming Anti-Inflammatory Foods**: An anti-inflammatory eating plan, like the Mediterranean diet, can help manage hypothyroidism. This diet focuses on plant-based foods, fish, seafood, whole grains, nuts, and seeds.
6. **Regular Consumption of Seafood and Seaweed**: These are excellent sources of iodine, a mineral essential for thyroid health.
7. **Inclusion of Lean Meats, Nuts, Seeds, and Leafy Greens**: These foods provide essential nutrients for thyroid function.
8. **Moderate Consumption of Dairy**: Dairy products, especially yogurt, provide probiotics and essential nutrients for thyroid health.
9. **Avoiding Excessive Intake of Goitrogens**: Certain foods contain substances called goitrogens that can interfere with thyroid function. These foods include broccoli, cabbage, and kale, but cooking these foods can inactivate the goitrogens.

Remember, everyone has different dietary needs and what works for one person may not work for another. It's important to consult with a healthcare provider or a dietitian before making significant changes to your diet.

Benefits of Hypothyroidism Diet

Incorporating a hypothyroidism diet can have several benefits for individuals with this condition, including:

1. **Improved Metabolism**: A well-balanced hypothyroidism diet can help improve metabolism, which is often slowed in individuals with hypothyroidism. This can lead to better energy levels and weight management.
2. **Enhanced Thyroid Function**: Consuming foods rich in iodine, selenium, and zinc can support thyroid hormone production and overall thyroid health, potentially improving symptoms of hypothyroidism.
3. **Weight Management**: By focusing on nutrient-dense, low-calorie foods, a hypothyroidism diet can help manage weight gain, a common issue for people with this condition.
4. **Reduced Inflammation**: Anti-inflammatory foods, such as fruits, vegetables, and lean proteins, can help reduce inflammation in the body, potentially alleviating some symptoms associated with hypothyroidism.
5. **Boosted Immune Function**: A diet rich in vitamins, minerals, and antioxidants can strengthen the immune system, promoting overall health and helping to fend off other conditions that can exacerbate hypothyroidism symptoms.

Following a hypothyroidism diet can not only improve symptoms but also contribute to overall health and well-being.

Disadvantages of Hypothyroidism Diet

While there are many benefits to following a hypothyroidism diet, it's important to be aware of any potential disadvantages, including:

- **Limited Food Options**: The need to avoid foods like soy-based products, cruciferous vegetables, and fatty foods can limit variety in the diet.
- **Risk of Nutrient Deficiencies**: Avoiding particular food groups may lead to a lack of certain nutrients if not properly balanced.
- **Increased Sensitivity to Gluten**: For some individuals with hypothyroidism, increased sensitivity to gluten may require the adoption of a gluten-free diet.
- **Difficulty in Balancing the Diet**: Striking a balance between foods that are generally healthy but potentially disruptive to thyroid function can be a challenge.

Through active management and treatment, the benefits of living with hypothyroidism can outweigh the disadvantages, leading to an improved overall quality of life.

5-Step Guide on How to Get Started with The Hypothyroidism Diet

Living with hypothyroidism can be challenging, but adjusting your diet can make a significant difference in managing your symptoms and enhancing your overall wellness. Here's a simple 5-step guide to help you begin a hypothyroidism-friendly diet.

Step 1: Engage Your Healthcare Provider

Before you embark on any significant alterations to your diet, it's vital that your first step is a thorough consultation with your healthcare provider. This could be your primary care doctor or a registered dietitian. These professionals possess a deep understanding of your unique health profile and are best equipped to provide guidance tailored to your specific needs.

In this consultation, they will likely review your current health status, your medical history, and the specifics of your hypothyroidism diagnosis. This information is crucial in creating a personalized dietary plan that addresses your individual requirements. Remember, what works for one person may not necessarily work for you; our bodies and health conditions are as unique as we are.

Your healthcare provider will also play a critical role in tracking your progress. As you make changes to your diet, they can monitor your body's response through regular check-ups and lab tests. This ongoing evaluation allows them to fine-tune your treatment plan if necessary, ensuring it remains effective over time.

Moreover, your healthcare provider can provide invaluable support throughout your journey. They can answer any questions you have, alleviate your concerns, and provide encouragement when you need it. They're your partner in this journey, providing expert guidance every step of the way.

So, before you head to the grocery store or start browsing new recipes, make sure your first stop is your healthcare provider's office. They'll equip you with the knowledge and tools you need to successfully manage your hypothyroidism through dietary changes.

Step 2: Adopt a Balanced Diet

Embracing a balanced diet is your next crucial step in managing hypothyroidism. This means diversifying your meals with a wide array of nutrient-rich foods from all the major food groups.

Start by incorporating lean proteins into your meals. Foods like chicken, turkey, fish, eggs, and legumes are excellent sources of protein. They not only help build and repair body tissues but also play a vital role in making hormones and enzymes.

Next, turn to whole grains. Foods such as brown rice, quinoa, oats, and whole grain bread are packed with fiber, helping you feel full longer and promoting healthy digestion. They also provide essential B vitamins that are necessary for energy production.

Fruits and vegetables should be a staple in your diet. They're loaded with vitamins, minerals, and antioxidants that boost your immune system, promote good heart health, and support overall well-being. Try to include a variety of colors on your plate to ensure you're getting a wide range of nutrients.

Don't forget about healthy fats. Foods like avocados, nuts, seeds, and olive oil provide monounsaturated and polyunsaturated fats that can help lower levels of "bad" LDL cholesterol and increase "good" HDL cholesterol. They also offer essential fatty acids that your body needs for brain function and cell growth.

These foods not only contribute to your general health but also play a key role in the proper functioning of your thyroid gland. Your thyroid needs certain nutrients, like iodine, selenium, and zinc, to produce thyroid hormones effectively.

A balanced diet ensures you're providing your body with these essential nutrients.

Remember, it's not just about what you eat, but also how you eat. Try to enjoy your meals without rushing, savor your food, and listen to your body's hunger and fullness cues. This mindful eating approach can enhance your relationship with food and promote better health.

So, as you embark on this journey, remember that variety is the spice of life and of a balanced diet. By incorporating a broad range of nutrient-rich foods into your meals, you're taking a significant step towards managing your hypothyroidism effectively.

Step 3: Moderate Consumption of Foods that Can Disrupt Thyroid Function

While maintaining a balanced diet is crucial, it's equally important to be aware of certain foods that can potentially interfere with your body's ability to utilize thyroid hormones.

Firstly, you might want to moderate your intake of soy products. Foods like tofu, soy milk, and edamame contain isoflavones, compounds that can affect the thyroid gland's ability to produce hormones, especially if you're not getting enough iodine in your diet. This doesn't mean you need to completely eliminate soy from your diet but consider enjoying these foods in moderation.

Next on the list are high-fiber foods. While fiber is essential for digestive health and can help control your weight, consuming an excessive amount can interfere with the absorption of thyroid medication. So, while you should still include fiber-rich foods in your diet, try to balance your intake throughout the day.

Certain cruciferous vegetables, including broccoli, cabbage, and kale, can also impact thyroid function when consumed in large quantities. These veggies contain substances known as goitrogens, which can disrupt the production of thyroid hormones. Again, you don't need to cut these out of your diet entirely – after all, they're packed with beneficial nutrients. However, try to consume them in reasonable amounts.

Remember, the goal isn't to banish these foods from your diet entirely. Each one still has its place in a balanced, nutritious eating plan. It's about creating a mindful approach towards your diet and understanding how different foods can affect your hypothyroidism. Moderation, as in many aspects of life, is key here.

By being aware of these potential food interactions and managing your intake appropriately, you'll be better equipped to support your thyroid health and overall well-being.

Step 4: Prioritize Hydration and Regular Physical Activity

Maintaining proper hydration and committing to regular exercise are two more significant steps you can take to manage hypothyroidism effectively. When it comes to hydration, aim to drink at least eight glasses of water per day. Staying well-hydrated isn't just about quenching your thirst; it also plays a vital role in numerous bodily functions. It aids in digestion, helps regulate body temperature, lubricates joints, and even impacts brain function.

Additionally, drinking enough water can help control hunger, which can be beneficial if weight management is part of your hypothyroidism treatment plan. Moving onto exercise, try to engage in at least 30 minutes of moderate-intensity physical activity on most days of the week. This could include activities like brisk walking, cycling, swimming, or even dancing.

Regular physical activity can help boost your metabolism, which tends to slow down with hypothyroidism, making weight loss more challenging. Exercise also has countless other benefits, from improving your mood and energy levels to promoting better sleep and cardiovascular health.

Remember, it's essential to find an exercise routine that you enjoy and fits into your lifestyle. This will make it easier for you to stick with it in the long term. And don't be too hard on yourself if you miss a day or two. The goal is consistency, not perfection.

In terms of hydration, if you're finding it difficult to consume eight glasses of water a day, try adding slices of lemon, cucumber, or fresh mint to your water for a flavorful twist. Or consider other hydrating foods like fruits and vegetables that have high water content.

Staying hydrated and exercising regularly are more than just general health advice—they're specific strategies that can help you manage hypothyroidism. With these habits, you're not just working towards better thyroid health, but you're also enhancing your overall well-being.

Step 5: Monitor Your Progress

The final step, but by no means the least important, is to continually monitor your progress. Remember, managing hypothyroidism isn't about reaching a final destination; it's an ongoing journey that requires consistent attention and care.

To start, make a habit of keeping track of your symptoms. This could include anything from fatigue and dry skin to sensitivity to cold and memory problems. Note any changes, no matter how subtle they may seem. This will allow you to better understand your body's responses and identify any patterns or triggers.

Alongside this, keep an eye on your energy levels. Hypothyroidism often leads to feelings of tiredness or lethargy, so any improvements in this area can be a positive sign that your management strategies are effective.

Weight changes are also worth monitoring. Hypothyroidism can often lead to weight gain, so if weight loss is part of your plan, tracking your progress can be motivating and informative. However, remember that health isn't solely defined by the number on the scale. Focus on how you feel overall, rather than getting too caught up in specific weight goals.

Regularly assessing your overall health can also provide valuable insights. Are you sleeping better? Do you have more mental clarity? Are your moods more stable? These kinds of questions can help assess the broader impact of your diet and treatment plan.

This ongoing monitoring is not just for your benefit—it's also crucial information for your healthcare provider. It can help them determine if your current diet and treatment plan are working effectively, or if any adjustments need to be made.

Remember, everyone's body is unique, and what works well for one person might not work as well for another. Always listen to your body and be prepared to make adjustments as necessary. You're the expert on your own body and its reactions, so don't hesitate to advocate for your needs and well-being.

Managing hypothyroidism is a dynamic process that requires ongoing attention and care. But with diligent monitoring and a willingness to adapt as needed, you can effectively manage your symptoms and enhance your overall health.

Foods to Eat

When following a hypothyroidism diet, it's important to focus on foods that can help support thyroid function and overall health. Here are some foods that are generally considered beneficial:

- **Iodine-rich foods**: Iodine is essential for the production of thyroid hormones. Foods rich in iodine include seaweed, fish, dairy products, and eggs.
- **Selenium-rich foods**: Selenium helps convert the thyroid hormone T4 into its active form, T3. Foods high in selenium include Brazil nuts, tuna, sardines, eggs, and legumes.
- **Zinc-rich foods**: Zinc also plays a crucial role in hormone production. Foods rich in zinc include oysters, beef, chicken, nuts, and whole grains.
- **Fiber-rich foods**: People with hypothyroidism often experience constipation. Fiber-rich foods can help improve digestion and alleviate this symptom. These include fruits, vegetables, and whole grains.

- **Healthy fats**: Healthy fats, found in avocados, olive oil, and nuts, can help maintain hormonal balance and reduce inflammation.
- **Protein-rich foods**: Protein helps transport thyroid hormone to all your tissues. Include a variety of protein sources in your diet such as lean meats, eggs, and legumes.
- **Antioxidant-rich foods**: These can help protect your thyroid gland from damage. Berries, bell peppers, and dark chocolate are all high in antioxidants.
- **Calcium and Vitamin D**: These nutrients are important for bone health, which can be compromised in people with hypothyroidism. Dairy products, fortified foods, fatty fish, and sunlight exposure can help meet these needs.

Remember, everyone's body reacts differently to different types of food. It's always a good idea to work with a healthcare provider or a dietitian to create a diet plan that suits your individual needs.

Foods to Avoid

While following a hypothyroidism diet, there are certain foods that you might want to avoid or limit, as they can interfere with your thyroid function or exacerbate your symptoms. Here are some of them:

1. **Soy**: Soy products like tofu, tempeh, edamame, and soy milk may interfere with the body's ability to use thyroid hormone. You don't necessarily need to avoid them completely but try not to consume them in large amounts.
2. **Cruciferous Vegetables**: Broccoli, cauliflower, kale, and other cruciferous vegetables can interfere with the production of thyroid hormone, particularly in people with an iodine deficiency. Cooking these vegetables can mitigate their goitrogenic properties.
3. **Gluten**: Some people with hypothyroidism, especially those with Hashimoto's thyroiditis, may be sensitive to gluten. If you notice your symptoms worsen after eating gluten, you might want to try a gluten-free diet.
4. **Fatty and Fried Foods**: These foods can inhibit the body's ability to absorb thyroid medication.
5. **Sugar**: People with hypothyroidism often have a slower metabolism, which can make it easy to put on weight. Limiting your sugar intake can help you maintain a healthy weight and keep your blood sugar levels stable.
6. **Excess Fiber**: While fiber is good for digestion, too much of it can interfere with your body's ability to absorb thyroid medication.
7. **Alcohol and Caffeine**: These can both interfere with the thyroid gland and should be consumed in moderation.

Remember, everyone's body reacts differently, and these are general guidelines rather than hard rules. Always consult with your healthcare provider or a dietitian for personalized advice.

Sample Meal Plan

Day 1

Breakfast

- Cheese Blintzes with Blackberries*
- Herbal Tea

Morning Snack

- Yoghurt with Mango Bits
- Plain Water

Lunch

- Moroccan-Style Chicken*
- Butternut Squash with Cinnamon*
- Water with Orange Slices

Afternoon Snack

- Liver Detox Shake*

Dinner

- Broiled Salmon with Dill
- Apple and Carrot Soup

- Plain Water

Day 2

Breakfast
- French Toast with Pear Slices
- Plain Water

Morning Snack
- Unsalted Almonds and Pecans
- Plain Water

Lunch
- Brown Rice with Tomato and avocado*
- Chicken Breast with Dijon Mustard
- Water with Cucumber Slices

Afternoon Snack
- Green Monster Smoothie*

Dinner
- Smoked Salmon and Watercress Salad
- Stuffed Mushrooms with Tapenade
- Plain Water

Day 3

Breakfast
- Granola with Apple, Banana, and Walnuts
- Lemon Tea

Morning Snack
- Cucumbers with Hummus
- Water with Lemon Slices

Lunch
- Angel Hair Pasta*
- Salmon Bruschetta

Afternoon Snack
- Pomegranate and Strawberry Parfait
- Plain Water

Dinner
- Honey Glazed Tuna
- Green Beans with Tomatoes
- Plain Water

Day 4

Breakfast
- Greek-Style Hash with California Sweet Potatoes*
- Plain Water

Morning Snack

- Turkey Ham Roll-ups
- Plain Water

Lunch

- Grapefruit and Crabmeat Salad
- Stuffed Eggplant
- Water with Lemon Slices

Afternoon Snack

- Orange Wheat Muffins
- Plain Water

Dinner

- Mackerel with Steamed Vegetables
- French Onion Soup
- Plain Water

Day 5

Breakfast

- Breakfast Smoothie

Morning Snack

- Unsalted Pumpkin Seeds
- Plain Water

Lunch

- Ginger-Chicken Noodle Soup*
- Grilled Eggplant
- Water with Lime Slices

Afternoon Snack

- French Crepes with Strawberries
- Plain Water

Dinner

- Pistachio Salmon*
- Pasta with Vegetables and Sun-Dried Tomatoes
- Plain Water

Day 6

Breakfast

- Rye Bread with Salmon and Cream Cheese
- Green Tea

Morning Snack

- Hard-boiled egg with Iodized Salt
- Plain Water

Lunch

- Smoky Stuffed Peppers*
- Bean Soup*

- Plain Water

Afternoon Snack

- Cherry Compote with Vanilla Ice Cream
- Plain Water

Dinner

- Herbed Chicken
- Kale Salad*
- Water with Lemon Slices

Day 7

Breakfast

- Scrambled Eggs with Caramelized Onions and Shiitake Mushrooms
- English Tea*

Morning Snack

- Oatmeal Cookies
- Plain Water

Lunch

- Polish-Style Beet Soup*
- Roasted Chicken Breast*
- Plain Water

Afternoon Snack
- Celery Sticks with Guacamole
- Water with Apple Slices

Dinner
- Tomato, Basil, and Mozzarella Salad
- Tuna with Balsamic Vinegar
- Plain Water

Remember, you are not required to follow this exact meal plan. However, you should observe the guiding principles of the hypothyroidism diet given earlier. As long as you abide by those guidelines, feel free to alter the recipes according to your personal preferences, or even insert your favorite recipes into the meal plan.

Tips to Implement Your Meal Plan

To keep you from suffering from the effects of hypothyroidism, here are some tips to help you implement your meal plan successfully:

Avoid Overcooking Your Food for Better Digestion

Overcooking your food, whether it's meat, vegetables, or grains, can sometimes make them tougher to digest. This is because the process of overcooking can break down the natural enzymes found in these foods that aid digestion. Additionally, overcooking can lead to a reduction in the nutrient content of the food, making it less beneficial for your health.

However, it's important to note that this doesn't mean you should switch entirely to a raw food diet. While raw foods are packed with enzymes and nutrients, they also contain fibers that can be difficult for some people's digestive systems to handle. Certain raw vegetables, for instance, have tough, fibrous structures that can be challenging to break down during digestion.

So, what's the solution? The key lies in finding a balance in the way you prepare your food to ensure it's easily digestible, while still retaining its nutritional value.

Take carrots, for example. Rather than consuming them raw or boiling them until they turn mushy, try blanching or steaming them for around 5 minutes. This method of cooking helps to soften the fibrous content, making it easier to digest, while still preserving most of the nutrients. You'll know you've got it right when your carrots retain a slight crunch—they shouldn't be too hard or too mushy.

This approach isn't just for carrots but can be applied to other vegetables like broccoli, cauliflower, and bell peppers. The goal is to cook these foods just enough to make them easier on your digestive system, without losing their nutritional benefits.

Furthermore, when it comes to grains and meats, consider methods like baking, grilling, or roasting instead of deep frying. These cooking techniques can help retain the food's natural enzymes and nutrients while making them easier to digest.

While it's essential to cook your food to make it safe for consumption, overcooking can make digestion more difficult and reduce the food's nutritional value. Striking a balance in your cooking methods can help ensure your food is not only delicious but also beneficial for your digestive health.

Take deep breaths before eating

In our fast-paced world, it's all too common to eat while feeling stressed, rushed, or distracted. However, this approach can lead to digestive issues like bloating, flatulence, and indigestion. That's why it's crucial to create a calm, relaxed environment for your body before you even begin your meal. One effective way to achieve this is through deep breathing exercises.

Deep breathing, also known as diaphragmatic breathing, involves fully engaging the stomach, abdominal muscles, and diaphragm when breathing. This type of breathing slows the heartbeat, can lower or stabilize blood pressure, and promotes better oxygen flow to our muscles and organs, including the digestive system.

To start, find a comfortable, quiet place to sit down. Once you're settled, begin by taking 10 deep, deliberate breaths. Inhale slowly through your nose, allowing your stomach to expand as you fill your lungs with air. Then, gently exhale through your mouth, releasing the air steadily and slowly.

For optimal results, aim for each inhale to last around 7 seconds, and each exhale to last about 14 seconds. This 1:2 ratio of inhale to exhale helps to stimulate the body's relaxation response, leading to a state of physical and mental calmness.

Practicing this simple but powerful exercise before eating serves multiple purposes. Firstly, it can help to reduce stress levels, which in turn can lower the risk of stress-induced digestive problems. Secondly, deep breathing increases the supply of oxygen and blood flow in your body, which can aid and speed up the digestive process.

Remember, digestion begins even before you take your first bite of food. By preparing your body and mind through deep breathing, you're setting the stage for more efficient digestion and better overall health. So before you dig into your next meal, take a moment to breathe deeply, relax, and fully engage with the process of nourishing your body. You might be surprised at the difference it makes!

Chew your food well

Digestion is a complex process that begins in the mouth. When we chew our food, we're not just breaking it down into smaller, more manageable pieces. We're also kick-starting the digestive process by mixing the food with saliva, which contains enzymes that begin the breakdown of food into a form your body can absorb and use.

Chewing well is an important but often overlooked aspect of good digestion. It's not just about making swallowing easier; it's about giving your digestive system a head start. The more thoroughly you chew your food, the less work your stomach has to do to break it down, which can reduce the risk of indigestion and other digestive issues.

Experts suggest that the optimal number of chews per bite of food is between 25 to 30. This might sound like a lot, especially if you're used to eating quickly. But taking the time to chew your food properly can make a significant difference to your digestive health.

To help build this habit, try counting your chews the next time you eat. This will give you a sense of how thoroughly you're currently chewing your food. If you find that you're falling short of the recommended 25 to 30 chews, make a conscious effort to slow down and chew each mouthful more thoroughly before swallowing.

It's also worth noting that chewing food thoroughly has other benefits too. It can help to improve the taste of your food, as it gives the flavors more time to spread across your palate. Additionally, it can help you to eat less, as it takes longer to eat, which can give your brain more time to realize that you're full.

So, the next time you sit down for a meal, remember to slow down, savor each bite, and chew thoroughly. Your digestive system will thank you!

Drink more water between your meals

Water is essential in the production of digestive fluids, such as amylase—an enzyme produced in the mouth—and hydrochloric acid in the stomach. These fluids, among others, are all affected by hypothyroidism, too.

Drinking more water in between meals would help in boosting the production of these digestive fluids. Take note that you should be drinking more between your meals, not during your meals. Doing the latter would actually hamper the digestive process since your drink would dilute the enzymes and acids needed to break down the food you are eating.

Rather than gulping down your drink during a meal, stick to taking little sips every now and then. Do not try to wash your food down with your drink. Just drink enough to rinse the flavor out of your mouth, or just to savor the taste of your beverage.

Move around after eating

There's a common perception that the primary benefit of physical activity after a meal is to burn calories. While it's true that moving around can help with calorie burning and weight management, there's another significant advantage that often goes overlooked – improved digestion.

Our digestive system relies on a series of coordinated muscle contractions, known as peristalsis, to move food through the digestive tract. Light physical activity after a meal, such as walking or gentle stretching, can stimulate this process and aid in the efficient movement of food along the digestive tract and intestines.

This can be particularly beneficial for people with conditions that slow down the digestive process, such as hypothyroidism. Hypothyroidism can reduce the motility rate of your digestive system, leading to symptoms like constipation, bloating, and abdominal discomfort. Engaging in light physical activity after meals can help to counteract this sluggishness, promoting better digestive health.

That said, it's important to keep the intensity of post-meal activities moderate. High-intensity workouts immediately after eating can divert blood flow away from the digestive system to the muscles, which can impede digestion rather than aid it. Gentle activities like walking, light yoga, or simple stretching exercises are typically more suitable.

So next time you finish a meal, consider taking a leisurely stroll or doing some light stretching. Not only can this help to manage your calorie intake, but it can also promote healthier, more efficient digestion. Remember, digestion doesn't just happen in the stomach—you can play an active role in supporting this vital process.

Sample Recipes

As indicated in Chapter 4 of this guide, here are the recipes of some items included in the sample 7-day meal plan for the hypothyroidism diet. Given below are the exact ingredients and procedures that must be followed to recreate these meals on your own. You may adjust the quantities depending on the number of servings that you wish to make.

Moroccan-Style Chicken

Ingredients:

- 2 lbs. chicken (any combination of breast halves, thighs, and drumsticks), skin removed and finely shredded
- 2/3 cup orange juice
- 2 tablespoons honey
- 1 tablespoon fresh ginger
- 1 tablespoon extra-virgin olive oil
- 1 teaspoon ground cumin
- 1 teaspoon paprika
- ½ teaspoon ground coriander
- ¼ teaspoon red pepper, crushed
- 1/8 teaspoon salt

Procedure:

1. Place all chicken cuts in a large re-sealable bag that is set in a deep dish container.
2. In a separate bowl, combine ½ cup orange juice, olive oil, ginger, crushed red pepper, cumin, coriander, paprika, and salt.
3. Pour the mixture over the chicken cuts inside the bag.
4. Seal the bag.
5. Turn the bag over to coat the chicken cuts with the marinade.

6. Store in the refrigerator for 24 hours, or at least 4 hours. Turn the bag over occasionally for even marinating of the chicken.
7. Drain the chicken, and discard the remaining marinade.
8. Set up the grill for indirect grilling.
9. Check if the heat above the pan you are using is only medium heat.
10. Place the drip pan under the grill rack.
11. Grease lightly the grill rack.
12. Place the chicken on the rack, skinned sides up.
13. Cover the rack, and grill for 50 minutes to 1 hour, or until the chicken breasts have reached 170 0F (76.67 0C) and the chicken thighs and drumsticks have reached 180 0F (82.22 0C).

Yield: 4 to 6 servings

Tip: For better taste, occasionally brush the chicken cuts with honey during the last 10 minutes of grilling.

Green Monster Smoothie

Ingredients:

- 1 small banana, frozen
- 2 cups baby spinach
- 2 cups ice, crushed
- 1 cup almond milk, unsweetened
- 1 scoop vanilla protein powder
- 1 tablespoon chia seeds

Procedure:

1. Put all the ingredients in a blender.
2. Blend until a smooth texture has been achieved.

Yield: 1 to 2 servings

Angel Hair Pasta

Ingredients:

- 4 ounces angel hair pasta, cooked according to the directions indicated in the packaging
- ½ lb. shrimps, peeled
- 1 green bell pepper, chopped
- 1 zucchini, chopped
- 1/3 cup pesto sauce, pre-made or homemade
- 2 tablespoons extra-virgin olive oil

Procedure:

1. Pour 1 tablespoon olive oil into a medium-sized skillet.
2. Cook shrimp in the skillet until they have turned brown.
3. Remove cooked shrimp from the pan.
4. Cook the bell pepper and zucchini in the skillet until they have become tender.
5. In a bowl, toss the pasta, shrimp, and vegetables with the pesto sauce.
6. Serve immediately.

Yield: 2 servings

Tip: When cooking the shrimp, avoid stirring them too much. Otherwise, you will not get a crust.

Greek-style hash with California Sweet Potatoes

Ingredients:

- 4 cups California sweet potatoes, shredded
- 4 cups baby spinach, chopped
- 4 large eggs
- 4 ounces feta cheese, crumbled
- 1 medium onion, finely chopped
- 1 tablespoon dried Greek seasoning
- Freshly ground black pepper, to taste
- Fresh oregano (optional; as garnish)

Procedure:

1. Heat the olive oil in a 12-inch skillet over medium heat setting.
2. Add the shredded sweet potatoes.
3. Toss in oil to coat.
4. Cook for around 5 minutes while stirring regularly to avoid burning the sweet potatoes.
5. Add the chopped onions.
6. Cook for another 4 minutes.
7. Add the chopped spinach.
8. Cook for 1 to 2 minutes, or until the leaves have wilted.
9. Stir in the Greek seasoning, salt, and black pepper to taste.

10. Spread the vegetables evenly on the pan.
11. Make 4 holes in the vegetables.
12. Crack 1 egg in each of the holes.
13. Cook for about 2 minutes.
14. Cover the pan with its lid.
15. Cook for another 3 minutes, or until eggs have been cooked according to your preference.
16. Remove the pan from the heat.
17. Top with crumbled feta cheese.
18. Garnish with fresh oregano.
19. Divide into 4, and serve immediately.

Yield: 4 servings

Tip: For better results, use a cast-iron skillet.

Pistachio Salmon

Ingredients:

- 6 salmon fillets (around 6 ounces each)
- 1 cup unsalted pistachios, chopped
- ½ cup packed brown sugar
- 3 tablespoons lemon juice
- 1 teaspoon dill weed
- A pinch of black pepper, to taste

Procedure:

1. Preheat the oven to 425 0F (218.33 0C).
2. Place the salmon fillets on a lightly greased 13-by-9-inch baking dish.
3. Combine the pistachios, brown sugar, lemon juice, dill weed, and black pepper in a separate bowl.
4. Spoon over the mixture over the salmon fillets.
5. Bake without cover for about 12 to 15 minutes, or until the salmon is easily flaking when checked with a fork.

Yield: 6 servings

Ginger-Chicken Noodle Soup

Ingredients:

- 1 lb. chicken thighs, skin and bones removed, cut into 1-inch pieces
- 3 cans of low-sodium chicken broth (around 14 ounces each)
- 2 medium carrots, sliced into bite-sized sticks
- 6 ounces pea pods, frozen, thawed, and sliced in half diagonally
- 2 ounces rice noodles, dried
- 1 cup water
- 2 tablespoons rice vinegar
- 1 tablespoon low-sodium soy sauce
- 1 tablespoon cooking oil
- 2 ½ teaspoons fresh ginger, minced
- Ground black pepper to taste

Procedure:

1. Using a Dutch oven, cook the chicken thighs—half a batch at a time—in hot oil until they have browned.
2. Drain all the chicken fat.
3. Place back the chicken thighs into the Dutch oven.
4. Add the carrot sticks, chicken broth, water, vinegar, soy sauce, minced ginger, and black pepper, to taste.
5. Bring to a boil.
6. Reduce the heat to low.

7. Simmer with the lid on for 20 minutes.
8. Bring to another boil.
9. Add the rice noodles.
10. Simmer without the lid for about 8 to 10 minutes, or until the noodles have become tender.
11. Add the pea pods during the last 1 to 2 minutes of cooking.
12. Serve immediately with soy sauce on the side, if desired.

Yield: *4 to 6 servings*

Smoky Stuffed Peppers

Ingredients:

- 6 large bell peppers, any color, tops, and seeds removed
- 12 ounces Italian turkey sausage, hot links, casing removed
- 4 medium plum tomatoes, chopped
- 1 ½ cups low-sodium chicken broth
- 2 cups brown rice, instant
- 1 cup fresh basil, chopped
- 1 cup smoked mozzarella cheese, finely shredded, divided

Procedure:

1. Place the rack in the upper third of the oven.
2. Preheat the broiler.
3. Arrange the bell peppers—cut side down—on a large microwaveable dish.
4. Fill the dish with ½ inch water.
5. Cover the dish with its lid.
6. Place the covered dish into the microwave.
7. Cook on high heat setting for about 7 to 10 minutes, or until the peppers have softened.
8. Drain the excess water.
9. Transfer bell peppers into a roasting pan.

10. In a large non-stick skillet, break sausage into small pieces using a wooden spoon.
11. Cook sausage in the skillet using medium-high heat for about 5 minutes, or until sausage pieces have been cooked through.
12. Stir in chicken broth, tomatoes, and rice.
13. Bring to a simmer by increasing the heat to high.
14. Cover the skillet with a lid.
15. Reduce the heat to medium-low
16. Cook the rice for about 5 minutes, or until it has softened while remaining moist.
17. Remove from heat, but keep the lid on.
18. Let it stand for 5 minutes, or until the rice has absorbed the remaining liquid.
19. Stir in the chopped basil, and half of the cheese into the rice.
20. Spoon the rice mixture into each of the bell pepper cups.
21. Top each filled bell pepper with the remaining cheese.
22. Broil bell peppers for 2 to 3 minutes, or until the cheese on top has melted.
23. Serve immediately.

Yield: *6 servings*

Tip #1: You can speed up the process of preparing the bell peppers by blanching them first in the microwave.

Tip #2: To further shorten the cooking time, you may consider using instant brown rice for this recipe.

Tip #3: For better results, select bell peppers that can stand upright on their own.

Tip #4: To boost the flavor, you may replace the smoked mozzarella cheese with smoked cheddar cheese or gouda cheese.

Kale Salad

Ingredients:

- 1 cup kale, chopped
- 6 artichokes or hearts of palm, diced
- 6 radishes, chopped
- 1 lemon, juiced
- ¼ cup coconut flakes
- ¼ cup coconut milk

Procedure:

1. Place all of the ingredients together in a bowl.
2. Toss well.
3. Serve chilled.

Yield: 1 to 2 servings

Polish-Style Beet Soup

Ingredients:

- 2 cups red beets, chopped
- 1 cup sweet potatoes, chopped
- 1 cup carrots, chopped
- 1 cup parsnip, chopped
- 1 medium onion, chopped
- 6 cups bone broth
- 2 bay leaves
- ½ teaspoon garlic powder
- 1 tablespoon lemon juice or apple cider vinegar, to taste
- A pinch of sea salt or pink Himalayan sea salt, to taste
- A pinch of ground black pepper (optional)
- 3 allspice berries (optional)

Procedure:

1. In a large stockpot, place the beets, sweet potatoes, carrots, parsnip, onion, bone broth, bay leaves, and garlic powder.
2. Bring it to a boil.
3. Reduce the heat to a simmer.
4. Add 1 tablespoon of lemon juice or apple cider vinegar.
5. Simmer for 40 minutes, or until all the vegetables have been cooked through.

6. Sprinkle with salt, pepper, and additional lemon juice or apple cider vinegar, according to your taste.
7. Serve immediately.

Yield: 6 servings

Tip #1: You can bring out a more vibrant shade of red from the beets if you would lemon juice.

Tip #2: If you had not chopped the vegetables before cooking, you may mash them after they have been cooked through. You may use a potato masher or a high-powered blender, in case you want a pureed soup. Be careful when blending hot liquids. Make sure that the top of the blender is properly vented to provide an outlet for the steam.

Brown Rice with Tomato and Avocado

Ingredients:

- 1 cup brown rice, cooked
- 15 cherry tomatoes
- 2 garlic cloves, minced
- 1 lemon, squeezed
- 1 avocado, sliced
- 1 tablespoon extra-virgin olive oil
- A few sprigs of cilantro

Procedure:

1. In a bowl, mix together the brown rice, cherry tomatoes, lemon juice, avocado slices, and cilantro.
2. Season with salt and black pepper according to taste.
3. Transfer to a flat plate.
4. Serve immediately.

Yield: 2 servings

Liver Detox Shake

Ingredients:

- 1 banana
- 1 apple
- 1 lemon, squeezed
- ½ cucumber
- 1 glass water
- ½ chili pepper (optional)
- 1 or more garlic cloves, according to preference (optional)

Procedure:

1. Place all ingredients into a blender.
2. Blend well until the texture has become smooth.
3. Pour into your preferred container.
4. Serve immediately.

Yield: 1 serving

Tip: Add your favorite fresh herbs, such as mint, cilantro, or parsley, for a little variety.

Cheese Blintzes with Blackberries

Ingredients:

For the Blintz Batter:

- 4 large eggs
- 1 cup milk
- 1 cup all-purpose flour
- Pinch of salt
- 2 tablespoons sugar
- Butter for frying

For the Cheese Filling:

- 1 cup ricotta cheese
- 1 cup cream cheese
- 1/4 cup sugar
- 1 teaspoon vanilla extract

For the Blackberry Sauce:

- 2 cups fresh blackberries
- 1/4 cup sugar
- 1 tablespoon lemon juice

Instructions:

1. Prepare the Blintz Batter: In a blender, combine the eggs, milk, flour, salt, and sugar. Blend until smooth. Let the batter rest for about 15 minutes.

2. Cook the Blintzes: Heat a small non-stick pan over medium heat. Melt a bit of butter in the pan, then pour in about 1/4 cup of the batter, swirling it around to evenly coat the bottom of the pan. Cook until the blintz is set and lightly golden on the bottom, then flip and cook for another minute. Repeat with the remaining batter.
3. Prepare the Cheese Filling: In a bowl, mix together the ricotta cheese, cream cheese, sugar, and vanilla extract until well combined.
4. Assemble the Blintzes: Place a spoonful of the cheese mixture in the center of each blintz. Fold the bottom edge towards the center, then fold in the sides and roll up the blintz, similar to a burrito.
5. Make the Blackberry Sauce: In a saucepan, combine the blackberries, sugar, and lemon juice. Cook over medium heat until the berries have broken down and the sauce has thickened.
6. Serve the Blintzes: Top the cheese blintzes with the blackberry sauce and serve immediately. Enjoy your homemade Cheese Blintzes with Blackberries!

Note: This recipe serves about 4 people. Adjust the ingredients proportionately based on your requirements.

English Tea

Ingredients:

- 1 tea bag or 1 teaspoon of loose-leaf black tea (per cup)
- Freshly boiled water
- Milk (optional)
- Sugar or honey (optional)

Instructions:

1. Boil the Water: Start by boiling fresh water in a kettle. The water should be heated until it reaches a rolling boil.
2. Prep Your Teapot or Cup: While your water is heating, if you're using a teapot, warm it up by rinsing it with hot water. If you're making tea in a cup, place your tea bag or loose-leaf tea (in a tea infuser) directly into the cup.
3. Steep the Tea: Once your water has reached a boil, pour it over the tea bag or tea leaves. Let the tea steep for about 3-5 minutes. For a stronger brew, let it steep a bit longer.
4. Remove the Tea Bag or Leaves: After the tea has steeped, remove the tea bag or infuser. Do not squeeze the tea bag as this can make the tea taste bitter.
5. Add Milk and Sweetener: If you like, add milk to your liking. Traditionally, English tea is served with a

splash of milk. You can also add sugar or honey to sweeten your tea.
6. Serve: Your English tea is now ready to enjoy. It's traditionally served with biscuits or scones on the side.

Tip: The key to a good cup of English tea is the quality of the tea you start with and using freshly boiled water. Enjoy your tea time!

Roasted Chicken Breast

Ingredients:

- 2 boneless, skin-on chicken breasts
- 2 tablespoons olive oil
- Salt and pepper to taste
- 1 teaspoon dried rosemary (or thyme, oregano, or your preferred herb)
- 2 cloves garlic, minced
- Juice of half a lemon

Instructions:

1. Preheat the Oven: Start by preheating your oven to 400°F (200°C).
2. Prepare the Chicken: Pat the chicken breasts dry with paper towels. This will help the skin get nice and crispy.
3. Season the Chicken: Rub the chicken breasts with olive oil, then season them generously with salt and pepper. Sprinkle the dried rosemary and minced garlic evenly over the chicken. Squeeze the lemon juice on top.
4. Roast the Chicken: Place the chicken breasts in a roasting pan or on a baking sheet. Roast in the preheated oven for about 20-25 minutes, or until the chicken is cooked through and the juices run clear. The

internal temperature should be at least 165°F (74°C) when measured with a meat thermometer.
5. Rest the Chicken: Once the chicken is done, let it rest for about 10 minutes before slicing. This allows the juices to redistribute throughout the chicken, making it more moist and flavorful.
6. Serve: Your Roasted Chicken Breast is now ready to enjoy. You can serve it with a side of vegetables, rice, or salad.

Tip: Cooking times can vary based on the size of the chicken breast and individual oven temperatures. Always ensure your chicken is thoroughly cooked before serving. Enjoy your meal!

Butternut Squash with Cinnamon

Ingredients:

- 1 medium-sized butternut squash
- 2 tablespoons of olive oil
- 2 teaspoons of ground cinnamon
- Salt and pepper to taste

Instructions:

1. Preheat your oven to 400°F (200°C). While the oven is heating, prepare your butternut squash.
2. Peel the butternut squash and cut it in half lengthwise. Scoop out the seeds and discard them (or save them for roasting later!).
3. Cut the butternut squash into 1-inch cubes. Try to make them as uniform as possible so they cook evenly.
4. Place the cubed butternut squash on a baking sheet. Drizzle the olive oil over the squash, ensuring all the pieces are lightly coated.
5. Sprinkle the ground cinnamon evenly over the butternut squash. Add salt and pepper to taste.
6. Toss the butternut squash to ensure all the pieces are evenly coated in the oil and spices.
7. Roast the butternut squash in the preheated oven for 25-30 minutes, or until the squash is tender and lightly browned. Halfway through the cooking time, stir the squash to ensure it cooks evenly.

8. Once done, remove the butternut squash from the oven and let it cool slightly before serving. Enjoy this delicious and healthy side dish!
9. Remember, this recipe is versatile, so feel free to add other spices or herbs if you wish!

Hearty Bean Soup

Ingredients:

- 2 cups dry mixed beans (or canned if you prefer)
- 1 large onion, chopped
- 2 carrots, chopped
- 2 celery stalks, chopped
- 3 cloves of garlic, minced
- 1 can diced tomatoes (14.5 oz)
- 6 cups of vegetable broth or water
- 1 teaspoon dried thyme
- 1 teaspoon dried rosemary
- Salt and pepper to taste
- 2 tablespoons olive oil

Instructions:

1. If you're using dry beans, soak them overnight in a large bowl of water. If you're using canned beans, rinse and drain them before use.
2. In a large pot, heat the olive oil over medium heat. Add the chopped onion, carrots, and celery. Sauté until the vegetables are softened, about 5 minutes.
3. Add the minced garlic to the pot and sauté for another minute until fragrant.
4. If you're using dry beans, drain them from their soaking water and add them to the pot. If you're using canned beans, add them now.

5. Add the canned tomatoes, vegetable broth or water, thyme, and rosemary to the pot. Stir everything together and bring the mixture to a simmer.
6. Reduce the heat to low and let the soup simmer for about 2 hours, or until the beans are cooked through and tender. If you're using canned beans, you only need to let it simmer for about 20-30 minutes.
7. Season the soup with salt and pepper to taste. You can also add more herbs or spices if you like.
8. Serve the bean soup hot, with a side of crusty bread if desired.

Conclusion

Congratulations! You've made it to the end of this comprehensive guide on diet management for hypothyroidism. By reaching this point, you've taken a big step towards understanding how your diet can influence your thyroid health, and that's something to be proud of.

Embarking on this journey is a testament to your commitment to better health. Remember, every small change you make, every new habit you form, brings you one step closer to managing your hypothyroidism effectively and enhancing your overall well-being.

Navigating through the world of dietary do's and don'ts can be a challenge, but you've already shown great initiative by seeking out information and taking steps to educate yourself. This guide has provided you with a roadmap to help manage your hypothyroidism through dietary changes. We've covered the importance of consuming nutrient-rich foods, moderating your intake of certain foods, staying hydrated, exercising regularly, and monitoring your progress.

But remember, this guide is just that—a guide. It's a starting point and a reference tool, but the real journey unfolds in your daily life, through the choices you make and the habits you cultivate. The key is to take things at your own pace and listen to your body. It's not about perfection, but about making consistent, sustainable changes that support your thyroid health.

Remember that managing hypothyroidism is a journey, not a destination. It's about understanding your body and learning how to best support it through nutrition and lifestyle choices. Some days will be easier than others, and that's okay. Celebrate your victories, no matter how small they may seem, and don't be too hard on yourself during the more challenging times.

Always keep in mind that everyone's experience with hypothyroidism is unique. What works for someone else may not work for you, and vice versa. It's all about finding the balance that works best for your body and your lifestyle.

And finally, remember that you're not alone in this journey. There's a whole community of people out there who understand what you're going through and are ready to offer support. Reach out, share your experiences, and learn from others. Together, we can make managing hypothyroidism less daunting and more manageable.

So here's to you, to the journey you've embarked on, and to the progress you'll undoubtedly make. You've taken the first step by educating yourself, and that's a significant achievement. Keep going, keep learning, and keep striving for better health. You've got this!

In conclusion, managing hypothyroidism is not just about taking medication—it's also about making informed dietary choices and leading a balanced lifestyle. This guide has equipped you with the knowledge and tools to do just that. So here's to your health and to taking control of your hypothyroidism—one healthy choice at a time!

FAQ

What foods are good for hypothyroidism?

A balanced diet rich in whole foods is beneficial for managing hypothyroidism. Foods high in selenium like Brazil nuts, tuna, and sardines, and foods high in iodine like seaweed, dairy products, and iodized salt can support thyroid health. Also, fruits, vegetables, lean proteins, and whole grains can contribute to overall well-being.

Are there any foods I should avoid with hypothyroidism?

While no food needs to be entirely eliminated, some foods may interfere with thyroid function or medication absorption. These include highly processed foods, excessive amounts of soy, and cruciferous vegetables like broccoli and cabbage if consumed in large quantities.

How can diet affect hypothyroidism?

Diet plays a crucial role in managing hypothyroidism. Certain nutrients, like iodine and selenium, are essential for thyroid function. Conversely, certain foods might interfere with thyroid hormone production or the absorption of thyroid medication.

Does gluten affect hypothyroidism?

Some research suggests that people with hypothyroidism, particularly those with Hashimoto's thyroiditis, may also have celiac disease or gluten sensitivity. In such cases, consuming gluten can trigger an immune response and potentially worsen hypothyroid symptoms.

Can a diet help manage hypothyroid symptoms?

Yes, a well-balanced diet can help manage hypothyroid symptoms. Consuming a variety of nutrient-rich foods can support general health and energy levels while avoiding certain foods can help prevent potential interference with thyroid function or medication.

Should I follow a specific diet plan for hypothyroidism?

There's no one-size-fits-all diet for hypothyroidism. However, eating a balanced diet rich in fruits, vegetables, lean protein, and whole grains can support overall health. It's also important to consume enough iodine and selenium, which are essential for thyroid function.

Can changing my diet cure hypothyroidism?

While a healthy diet can help manage symptoms and support thyroid health, it's not a cure for hypothyroidism. Hypothyroidism is a chronic condition that often requires lifelong treatment with thyroid hormone replacement medication. Always consult with your healthcare provider before making any significant changes to your diet or medication regimen.

References and Helpful Links

Rd, R. R. M. (2023, July 31). What's the best diet for hypothyroidism? Healthline. https://www.healthline.com/nutrition/hypothyroidism-diet

Hypothyroidism diet: Can certain foods increase thyroid function? (2023, August 18). Mayo Clinic. https://www.mayoclinic.org/diseases-conditions/hypothyroidism/expert-answers/hypothyroidism-diet/faq-20058554

Thompson, D., Jr. (2023, October 21). 9 Foods to Avoid with Hypothyroidism. EverydayHealth.com. https://www.everydayhealth.com/hs/thyroid-pictures/foods-to-avoid/

Hypothyroidism (underactive thyroid) - Symptoms and causes - Mayo Clinic. (2022, December 10). Mayo Clinic. https://www.mayoclinic.org/diseases-conditions/hypothyroidism/symptoms-causes/syc-20350284

Professional, C. C. M. (n.d.). Thyroid disease. Cleveland Clinic. https://my.clevelandclinic.org/health/diseases/8541-thyroid-disease

Facp, P. R. O. M. (n.d.). Hypothyroidism Treatment & management: Approach considerations, Hypothyroidism in pregnancy, Subclinical hypothyroidism. https://emedicine.medscape.com/article/122393-treatment

GoodRX - error. (n.d.-b). https://www.goodrx.com/conditions/hypothyroidism/nutrition-and-hypothyroidism

www.ingramcontent.com/pod-product-compliance
Lightning Source LLC
LaVergne TN
LVHW010429070526
838199LV00066B/5969